This journal belongs to

_____

_____

Copyright @2019 Marite Zen

All rights reserved. No part of this publication may be reproduced, distributed or transmitted in any means without the prior written permission of the Publisher.

Although every precaution has been taken to verify the accuracy of the information contained herein, the author and publisher assume no responsibility for any errors or omissions. The tips and strategies contained herein may not be applicable to your situation. No liability is assumed for damages that may result from the use of information contained within.

ISBN: 9781070351285

CONTENTS

1. Eating tips for endometriosis

2. Daily tracker log sheets

3. Pain level trends

4. My favourite recipes

How Does it Work?

In recent years, there has been increasing awareness around endometriosis. Considering how this condition usually takes several years only to be diagnosed, this is already a big step forward.

What is still missing, however, is an effective and holistic therapeutic approach that is not merely based on prescription of long-term drugs or on invasive surgery, and on the other hand will not leave women on their own researching information around alternative and integrating treatments.

As an endometriosis sufferer, I have often noticed, when learning about other women's experiences, how an actual improvement in symptoms occurs when the person's attitude towards the disease changes; that is when one stops blindly surrendering to doctors or other healing figures, to get into a path of self-reflection and connection with the deeper causes behind the physical discomfort.

This occurs when women develop (or rather regain) the ability to listen to their own bodies and emotions, in order to take the necessary caring measures, be it by taking medicines or by practising yoga and meditation.

This journal has been designed to help women suffering from endometriosis take their health back in control by focusing their awareness on the body's pain symptoms and relieving these, especially through daily diet.

The connection between endometriosis and nutrition is in fact increasingly being discussed, still with many different approaches and beliefs. By tracking your daily food intake and pain symptoms, this log journal will give you the means to pinpoint potential trigger foods based on your own experience.

As mentioned, there are many suggested diets and nutrition protocols for endometriosis. In the following section, you can find a summary of some of the main guidelines – see also the overview available at:

https://endometriosis.net/living/what-to-eat/

At the end of the journal, you will also find a section where you can write down your personalised recipes which are most suitable and appetising for you.

Hugs,

Marite

Eating Tips for Endometriosis

--> Read and memorise the main diet guidelines suitable for endometriosis.

--> Try to stick to these as much as possible.

Foods to Increase

High-Fibre Foods

High fibrous foods are known to lower estrogen levels and stabilise hormonal activity.

- **Vegetables and fruits rich in fibre** - These contain flavonoids, carotenoids, and vitamins A, C, and E. Flavonoids and carotenoids are antioxidants that will reduce oxidative stress and inflammation in the body.

- **Whole grains** are grains that are not processed where their outer kernel has not been removed. These retain much of their nutritional value and fibrous content.

  - ☐ Oatmeal
  - ☐ Whole cornmeal
  - ☐ Quinoa
  - ☐ Barley
  - ☐ Whole rye
  - ☐ Brown rice

- **Beans and legumes** - these are full of magnesium, potassium, and soluble fibre. They also have a low glycemic index, which means they don't raise blood sugar levels and reduce inflammation.

  - ☐ Lentils
  - ☐ Chickpeas
  - ☐ Black beans

Omega 3 and Omega 6

Omega-3 fatty acids are polyunsaturated fatty acids (PUFA) which are famous for their cardio-protective effects.

They reduce triglyceride levels in the body, lower blood pressure, and also prevent deposition of fat in blood vessels.

- ☐ Nuts & Seeds
- ☐ Flax seeds
- ☐ Chia seeds

- ☐ Olive oli
- ☐ Coconut oil

- ☐ Oily fish (mackarel, sardines)
- ☐ Salmon
- ☐ Tuna

The benefits of Omega-6 are similar to those of Omega-3. However, some studies suggest that excessive consumption of Omega-6 fatty acids increases the levels of pro-inflammatory substances in the body. Therefore, it is essential to balance out Omega-6 and Omega-3 levels in the body.

Vegetable oils

- ☐ Corn oil
- ☐ Evening primrose oil
- ☐ Sunflower oil

Nuts

- ☐ Walnuts
- ☐ Almonds
- ☐ Pine nuts

- ☐ Vegetable sprouts

Foods to Limit

Wheat & Dairy

Wheat and dairy both contain carbohydrates that are difficult to digest and have the tendency to cause abdominal bloating; this can in turn increase the severity of pain in endometriosis.

These foods also contain phytic acid, a substance that prevents the absorption of iron, zinc, and calcium; leading to mineral deficiencies.

- ☐ Bread
- ☐ Pasta
- ☐ Pastries
- ☐ Baked products
- ☐ Milk
- ☐ Cheese
- ☐ Cream
- ☐ Butter

Red Meat

Red meat and processed meat are high in saturated fats and cholesterol.

They promote inflammatory processes in the body, increase the total body fat content, and may aggravate the symptoms of endometriosis.

- ☐ Beef
- ☐ Veal
- ☐ Pork
- ☐ Cured meat
- ☐ Frankfurters

Some meats may also contain hormones which can further lead to hormonal imbalance. For this reason, it is always better to opt for grass-fed lean meats, such as chicken and turkey.

Foods to Avoid

Sugars, Refined Carbohydrates & Trans fats

It is best to avoid foods that increase inflammation since they can worsen the symptoms of endometriosis; these include foods high in trans-fats, refined carbohydrates, fried food, and sugars.

Consumption of these food groups will also lead to hormonal imbalance and cause bloating, which can further increase abdominal and pelvic pain.

- ☐ Snacks
- ☐ Biscuits
- ☐ Sugary drinks
- ☐ Refined sugars
- ☐ Margarine
- ☐ White flour products

Soy Products

Foods containing soy are phytoestrogens, which can contribute to natural oestrogen production. The consumption of such foods may lead to hormonal imbalance and worsen the pain or cause irregular menstrual cycles.

- ☐ Edameme
- ☐ Seitan
- ☐ Tofu
- ☐ Soy sauce

Alcohol, Coffee and Energy drinks

Recommended Supplements

Vitamin D

Low levels of Vitamin D are often correlated with endometriosis, as well as with presence of ovarian cysts. Vitamin D is known to reduce inflammation and has immunoprotective effects. Supplementing one's diet with vitamin D will not only decrease the severity of endometriosis-related pain, but will also benefit general bone health.

Curcumin

Curcumin is a natural phytochemical which can be extracted from turmeric. Well known for its anti-inflammatory properties, this supplement can aid in mitigating symptoms of endometriosis thanks to its anti-inflammatory and anti-oxidative properties.

Furthermore, this substance intercepts the attachment of endometrial cells to ectopic sites by inhibiting the production of substances that regulate attachments and adhesions.

It prevents the formation of new blood vessels to the ectopic endometrial tissue, thereby reducing blood supply and blocking the growth of this tissue.

Probiotics

Probiotics help with gut health by promoting the growth of healthy gut flora and assisting with digestion. Gut health and endometriosis are often connected; when gut health is maintained, the severity of endometriosis pain can also be reduced.

Foods containing probiotics are foods such as yoghurt, yoghurt drinks, fermented foods and kombucha. Probiotics can also be consumed as supplements.

DIM

Diindolylmethane (DIM) is a bioactive food compound found in cruciferous vegetables (such as broccoli, bok choy, cabbage, cauliflower, Brussel sprouts, collard, and kale). The bioactive compounds released upon the consumption of cruciferous vegetables are metabolized into intermediates, one of which is DIM.

DIM has anticancer, anti-inflammatory, and anti-oxidant effects. It can modulate the effects of estrogen by preventing the activity of the enzyme which is responsible for estrogen metabolism.

Because DIM maintains hormonal balance, it generally helps in:

- Lowering the risk of hormonal acne
- Preventing breast cancer
- Decreasing estrogen levels in estrogen-dominant conditions (including fibroids and endometriosis)

Vitamin B6

Vitamin B6 breaks down and metabolizes estrogen. This will help in reducing pelvic pain and regulate menstrual cycles.

Vitamin B6 is also known to reduce symptoms of Premenstrual Syndrome (PMS).

Daily Tracker Log Sheets

--> Fill in the different sections of the daily log sheet and give an overall score of your pain symptoms - 0 being no pain and 10 very high levels of pain and discomfort.

DAILY TRACKER

Date: _____

(M) (T) (W) (T) (F) (S) (S)

Menstrual
cycle day _____

Breakfast
_____
_____

Supplements:
_____
_____

Lunch:
_____
_____

Medicines:
_____
_____

Dinner:
_____
_____

Pain Assessment

Pelvic	0	1	2	3	4	5	6	7	8	9	10
Abdominal	0	1	2	3	4	5	6	7	8	9	10
Rectal	0	1	2	3	4	5	6	7	8	9	10
Musculo skeletal	0	1	2	3	4	5	6	7	8	9	10
Sexual	0	1	2	3	4	5	6	7	8	9	10

Notes: _____
_____
_____

Overall score of the day

DAILY TRACKER

Date: _____

(M) (T) (W) (T) (F) (S) (S)

Menstrual cycle day _____

Breakfast
_____
_____

Lunch:
_____
_____

Dinner:
_____
_____

Supplements: _____
_____
_____

Medicines:
_____
_____

Pain Assessment

Pelvic	0	1	2	3	4	5	6	7	8	9	10
Abdominal	0	1	2	3	4	5	6	7	8	9	10
Rectal	0	1	2	3	4	5	6	7	8	9	10
Musculo skeletal	0	1	2	3	4	5	6	7	8	9	10
Sexual	0	1	2	3	4	5	6	7	8	9	10

Notes: _____
_____
_____
_____

Overall score of the day

( )

DAILY TRACKER

Date: _____

Ⓜ Ⓣ Ⓦ Ⓣ Ⓕ Ⓢ Ⓢ

Menstrual cycle day _____

Breakfast
_____
_____

Lunch:
_____
_____

Dinner:
_____
_____

Supplements:
_____
_____

Medicines:
_____
_____

Pain Assessment

Pelvic	0	1	2	3	4	5	6	7	8	9	10
Abdominal	0	1	2	3	4	5	6	7	8	9	10
Rectal	0	1	2	3	4	5	6	7	8	9	10
Musculoskeletal	0	1	2	3	4	5	6	7	8	9	10
Sexual	0	1	2	3	4	5	6	7	8	9	10

Notes: _____
_____
_____
_____

Overall score of the day

DAILY TRACKER

Date: _____

(M) (T) (W) (T) (F) (S) (S)

Breakfast
_____
_____

Lunch:
_____
_____

Dinner:
_____
_____

Menstrual cycle day _____

Supplements:
_____
_____

Medicines:
_____
_____

Pain Assessment

Pelvic	0	1	2	3	4	5	6	7	8	9	10
Abdominal	0	1	2	3	4	5	6	7	8	9	10
Rectal	0	1	2	3	4	5	6	7	8	9	10
Musculo skeletal	0	1	2	3	4	5	6	7	8	9	10
Sexual	0	1	2	3	4	5	6	7	8	9	10

Notes: _____
_____
_____
_____

Overall score of the day

( )

DAILY TRACKER

Date: _____

(M) (T) (W) (T) (F) (S) (S)

Menstrual
cycle day _____

Breakfast
_____
_____

Lunch:
_____
_____

Dinner:
_____
_____

Supplements:
_____
_____

Medicines:
_____
_____

Pain Assessment

Pelvic	0	1	2	3	4	5	6	7	8	9	10
Abdominal	0	1	2	3	4	5	6	7	8	9	10
Rectal	0	1	2	3	4	5	6	7	8	9	10
Musculo skeletal	0	1	2	3	4	5	6	7	8	9	10
Sexual	0	1	2	3	4	5	6	7	8	9	10

Notes: _____
_____
_____

Overall score of the day

DAILY TRACKER

Date: _____

(M) (T) (W) (T) (F) (S) (S)

Breakfast
_____
_____

Lunch:
_____
_____

Dinner:
_____
_____

Menstrual cycle day _____

Supplements:
_____
_____

Medicines:
_____
_____

Pain Assessment

Pelvic	0	1	2	3	4	5	6	7	8	9	10
Abdominal	0	1	2	3	4	5	6	7	8	9	10
Rectal	0	1	2	3	4	5	6	7	8	9	10
Musculo skeletal	0	1	2	3	4	5	6	7	8	9	10
Sexual	0	1	2	3	4	5	6	7	8	9	10

Notes: _____
_____
_____
_____

Overall score of the day

( )

DAILY TRACKER

Date: _____

(M) (T) (W) (T) (F) (S) (S)

Breakfast
_____
_____

Lunch:
_____
_____

Dinner:
_____
_____

Menstrual cycle day _____

Supplements:
_____
_____

Medicines:
_____
_____

Pain Assessment

Pelvic	0	1	2	3	4	5	6	7	8	9	10
Abdominal	0	1	2	3	4	5	6	7	8	9	10
Rectal	0	1	2	3	4	5	6	7	8	9	10
Musculo skeletal	0	1	2	3	4	5	6	7	8	9	10
Sexual	0	1	2	3	4	5	6	7	8	9	10

Notes: _____
_____
_____

Overall score of the day

DAILY TRACKER

Date: _____

(M) (T) (W) (T) (F) (S) (S)

Breakfast
_____
_____

Lunch:
_____
_____

Dinner:
_____
_____

Menstrual cycle day _____

Supplements:
_____
_____

Medicines:
_____
_____

Pain Assessment

Pelvic	0	1	2	3	4	5	6	7	8	9	10
Abdominal	0	1	2	3	4	5	6	7	8	9	10
Rectal	0	1	2	3	4	5	6	7	8	9	10
Musculo skeletal	0	1	2	3	4	5	6	7	8	9	10
Sexual	0	1	2	3	4	5	6	7	8	9	10

Notes: _____
_____
_____
_____

Overall score of the day

( )

DAILY TRACKER

Date: _____

(M) (T) (W) (T) (F) (S) (S)

Menstrual
cycle day _____

Breakfast
_____
_____

Supplements:
_____
_____

Lunch:
_____
_____

Medicines:
_____

Dinner:
_____
_____

Pain Assessment

Pelvic	0	1	2	3	4	5	6	7	8	9	10
Abdominal	0	1	2	3	4	5	6	7	8	9	10
Rectal	0	1	2	3	4	5	6	7	8	9	10
Musculo skeletal	0	1	2	3	4	5	6	7	8	9	10
Sexual	0	1	2	3	4	5	6	7	8	9	10

Notes: _____
_____
_____
_____

Overall score of the day

DAILY TRACKER

Date: _____

M T W T F S S

Breakfast _____

_____

Menstrual cycle day _____

Supplements: _____

_____

Lunch: _____

_____

_____

_____

Dinner: _____

Medicines: _____

_____

_____

_____

Pain Assessment

Pelvic	0	1	2	3	4	5	6	7	8	9	10
Abdominal	0	1	2	3	4	5	6	7	8	9	10
Rectal	0	1	2	3	4	5	6	7	8	9	10
Musculo skeletal	0	1	2	3	4	5	6	7	8	9	10
Sexual	0	1	2	3	4	5	6	7	8	9	10

Notes: _____

_____

_____

_____

Overall score of the day

◯

DAILY TRACKER

Date: _____

M T W T F S S

Menstrual cycle day _____

Breakfast
_____
_____

Lunch:
_____
_____

Dinner:
_____
_____

Supplements:
_____
_____

Medicines:
_____
_____

Pain Assessment

Pelvic	0	1	2	3	4	5	6	7	8	9	10
Abdominal	0	1	2	3	4	5	6	7	8	9	10
Rectal	0	1	2	3	4	5	6	7	8	9	10
Musculo skeletal	0	1	2	3	4	5	6	7	8	9	10
Sexual	0	1	2	3	4	5	6	7	8	9	10

Notes: _____
_____
_____
_____

Overall score of the day

DAILY TRACKER

Date: _____

（M）（T）（W）（T）（F）（S）（S）

Breakfast
_____
_____

Lunch:
_____
_____

Dinner:
_____
_____

Menstrual
cycle day _____

Supplements:
_____
_____

Medicines:
_____
_____

Pain Assessment

| Pelvic | 0 | 1 | 2 | 3 | 4 | 5 | 6 | 7 | 8 | 9 | 10 |

| Abdominal | 0 | 1 | 2 | 3 | 4 | 5 | 6 | 7 | 8 | 9 | 10 |

| Rectal | 0 | 1 | 2 | 3 | 4 | 5 | 6 | 7 | 8 | 9 | 10 |

| Musculo skeletal | 0 | 1 | 2 | 3 | 4 | 5 | 6 | 7 | 8 | 9 | 10 |

| Sexual | 0 | 1 | 2 | 3 | 4 | 5 | 6 | 7 | 8 | 9 | 10 |

Notes: _____
_____
_____
_____

Overall score of the day

DAILY TRACKER

Date: _____

Ⓜ Ⓣ Ⓦ Ⓣ Ⓕ Ⓢ Ⓢ

Menstrual cycle day _____

Breakfast
_____
_____

Lunch:
_____
_____

Dinner:
_____
_____

Supplements:
_____
_____

Medicines:
_____
_____

Pain Assessment

Pelvic	0	1	2	3	4	5	6	7	8	9	10
Abdominal	0	1	2	3	4	5	6	7	8	9	10
Rectal	0	1	2	3	4	5	6	7	8	9	10
Musculo skeletal	0	1	2	3	4	5	6	7	8	9	10
Sexual	0	1	2	3	4	5	6	7	8	9	10

Notes: _____
_____
_____
_____

Overall score of the day

DAILY TRACKER

Date: _____

(M) (T) (W) (T) (F) (S) (S)

Breakfast
_____
_____

Lunch:
_____
_____

Dinner:
_____
_____

Menstrual cycle day _____

Supplements:
_____
_____

Medicines:
_____
_____

Pain Assessment

Pelvic	0	1	2	3	4	5	6	7	8	9	10
Abdominal	0	1	2	3	4	5	6	7	8	9	10
Rectal	0	1	2	3	4	5	6	7	8	9	10
Musculo skeletal	0	1	2	3	4	5	6	7	8	9	10
Sexual	0	1	2	3	4	5	6	7	8	9	10

Notes: _____
_____
_____
_____

Overall score of the day

DAILY TRACKER

Date: _____

Ⓜ Ⓣ Ⓦ Ⓣ Ⓕ Ⓢ Ⓢ

Menstrual cycle day _____

Breakfast
_____
_____

Lunch:
_____
_____

Dinner:
_____
_____

Supplements:
_____
_____

Medicines:
_____
_____

Pain Assessment

	0	1	2	3	4	5	6	7	8	9	10
Pelvic	0	1	2	3	4	5	6	7	8	9	10
Abdominal	0	1	2	3	4	5	6	7	8	9	10
Rectal	0	1	2	3	4	5	6	7	8	9	10
Musculoskeletal	0	1	2	3	4	5	6	7	8	9	10
Sexual	0	1	2	3	4	5	6	7	8	9	10

Notes: _____
_____
_____

Overall score of the day

DAILY TRACKER

Date: _____

(M) (T) (W) (T) (F) (S) (S)

Breakfast
_____
_____

Lunch:
_____
_____

Dinner:
_____
_____

Menstrual cycle day _____

Supplements:
_____
_____

Medicines:
_____
_____

Pain Assessment

| Pelvic | 0 | 1 | 2 | 3 | 4 | 5 | 6 | 7 | 8 | 9 | 10 |

| Abdominal | 0 | 1 | 2 | 3 | 4 | 5 | 6 | 7 | 8 | 9 | 10 |

| Rectal | 0 | 1 | 2 | 3 | 4 | 5 | 6 | 7 | 8 | 9 | 10 |

| Musculo skeletal | 0 | 1 | 2 | 3 | 4 | 5 | 6 | 7 | 8 | 9 | 10 |

| Sexual | 0 | 1 | 2 | 3 | 4 | 5 | 6 | 7 | 8 | 9 | 10 |

Notes: _____
_____
_____
_____

Overall score of the day

DAILY TRACKER

Date: _____

(M) (T) (W) (T) (F) (S) (S)

Breakfast
_____
_____

Lunch:
_____
_____

Dinner:
_____
_____

Menstrual cycle day _____

Supplements:
_____
_____

Medicines:
_____
_____

Pain Assessment

Pelvic	0	1	2	3	4	5	6	7	8	9	10
Abdominal	0	1	2	3	4	5	6	7	8	9	10
Rectal	0	1	2	3	4	5	6	7	8	9	10
Musculo skeletal	0	1	2	3	4	5	6	7	8	9	10
Sexual	0	1	2	3	4	5	6	7	8	9	10

Notes: _____
_____
_____

Overall score of the day

DAILY TRACKER

Date: _____

Ⓜ Ⓣ Ⓦ Ⓣ Ⓕ Ⓢ Ⓢ

Menstrual cycle day _____

Breakfast
_____
_____

Lunch:
_____
_____

Dinner:
_____
_____

Supplements:
_____
_____

Medicines:
_____
_____

Pain Assessment

	0	1	2	3	4	5	6	7	8	9	10
Pelvic	0	1	2	3	4	5	6	7	8	9	10
Abdominal	0	1	2	3	4	5	6	7	8	9	10
Rectal	0	1	2	3	4	5	6	7	8	9	10
Musculo skeletal	0	1	2	3	4	5	6	7	8	9	10
Sexual	0	1	2	3	4	5	6	7	8	9	10

Notes: _____
_____
_____
_____

Overall score of the day

DAILY TRACKER

Date: _____

Ⓜ Ⓣ Ⓦ Ⓣ Ⓕ Ⓢ Ⓢ

Menstrual cycle day _____

Breakfast
_____
_____

Lunch:
_____
_____

Dinner:
_____
_____

Supplements:
_____
_____

Medicines:
_____
_____

Pain Assessment

Pelvic	0	1	2	3	4	5	6	7	8	9	10
Abdominal	0	1	2	3	4	5	6	7	8	9	10
Rectal	0	1	2	3	4	5	6	7	8	9	10
Musculo skeletal	0	1	2	3	4	5	6	7	8	9	10
Sexual	0	1	2	3	4	5	6	7	8	9	10

Notes: _____
_____
_____
_____

Overall score of the day

DAILY TRACKER

Date: _____

Ⓜ Ⓣ Ⓦ Ⓣ Ⓕ Ⓢ Ⓢ

Menstrual cycle day _____

Breakfast
_____
_____

Supplements:
_____
_____

Lunch:
_____
_____

Medicines:
_____
_____

Dinner:
_____
_____

Pain Assessment

	0	1	2	3	4	5	6	7	8	9	10
Pelvic	0	1	2	3	4	5	6	7	8	9	10
Abdominal	0	1	2	3	4	5	6	7	8	9	10
Rectal	0	1	2	3	4	5	6	7	8	9	10
Musculo skeletal	0	1	2	3	4	5	6	7	8	9	10
Sexual	0	1	2	3	4	5	6	7	8	9	10

Notes: _____
_____
_____

Overall score of the day

DAILY TRACKER

Date: _____

(M) (T) (W) (T) (F) (S) (S)

Menstrual cycle day _____

Breakfast
_____
_____

Lunch:
_____
_____

Dinner:
_____
_____

Supplements:
_____
_____

Medicines:
_____
_____

Pain Assessment

| Pelvic | 0 | 1 | 2 | 3 | 4 | 5 | 6 | 7 | 8 | 9 | 10 |

| Abdominal | 0 | 1 | 2 | 3 | 4 | 5 | 6 | 7 | 8 | 9 | 10 |

| Rectal | 0 | 1 | 2 | 3 | 4 | 5 | 6 | 7 | 8 | 9 | 10 |

| Musculo skeletal | 0 | 1 | 2 | 3 | 4 | 5 | 6 | 7 | 8 | 9 | 10 |

| Sexual | 0 | 1 | 2 | 3 | 4 | 5 | 6 | 7 | 8 | 9 | 10 |

Notes: _____
_____
_____
_____

Overall score of the day

DAILY TRACKER

Date: _____

(M) (T) (W) (T) (F) (S) (S)

Breakfast
_____
_____

Lunch:
_____
_____

Dinner:
_____
_____

Menstrual cycle day _____

Supplements:
_____
_____

Medicines:
_____
_____

Pain Assessment

Pelvic	0	1	2	3	4	5	6	7	8	9	10
Abdominal	0	1	2	3	4	5	6	7	8	9	10
Rectal	0	1	2	3	4	5	6	7	8	9	10
Musculo skeletal	0	1	2	3	4	5	6	7	8	9	10
Sexual	0	1	2	3	4	5	6	7	8	9	10

Notes: _____
_____
_____

Overall score of the day

( )

DAILY TRACKER

Date: _____

M T W T F S S

Menstrual
cycle day _____

Breakfast
_____
_____

Lunch:
_____
_____

Dinner:
_____
_____

Supplements:
_____
_____

Medicines:
_____
_____

Pain Assessment

| Pelvic | 0 | 1 | 2 | 3 | 4 | 5 | 6 | 7 | 8 | 9 | 10 |

| Abdominal | 0 | 1 | 2 | 3 | 4 | 5 | 6 | 7 | 8 | 9 | 10 |

| Rectal | 0 | 1 | 2 | 3 | 4 | 5 | 6 | 7 | 8 | 9 | 10 |

| Musculo skeletal | 0 | 1 | 2 | 3 | 4 | 5 | 6 | 7 | 8 | 9 | 10 |

| Sexual | 0 | 1 | 2 | 3 | 4 | 5 | 6 | 7 | 8 | 9 | 10 |

Notes: _____
_____
_____

Overall score of the day

DAILY TRACKER

Date: _____

(M) (T) (W) (T) (F) (S) (S)

Menstrual cycle day _____

Breakfast
_____
_____

Lunch:
_____
_____

Dinner:
_____
_____

Supplements:
_____
_____

Medicines:
_____
_____

Pain Assessment

Pelvic	0	1	2	3	4	5	6	7	8	9	10
Abdominal	0	1	2	3	4	5	6	7	8	9	10
Rectal	0	1	2	3	4	5	6	7	8	9	10
Musculo skeletal	0	1	2	3	4	5	6	7	8	9	10
Sexual	0	1	2	3	4	5	6	7	8	9	10

Notes: _____
_____
_____
_____

Overall score of the day

DAILY TRACKER

Date: _____

(M) (T) (W) (T) (F) (S) (S)

Menstrual cycle day _____

Breakfast
_____
_____

Supplements:
_____
_____

Lunch:
_____
_____

Medicines:
_____

Dinner:
_____
_____

Pain Assessment

Pelvic	0	1	2	3	4	5	6	7	8	9	10
Abdominal	0	1	2	3	4	5	6	7	8	9	10
Rectal	0	1	2	3	4	5	6	7	8	9	10
Musculo skeletal	0	1	2	3	4	5	6	7	8	9	10
Sexual	0	1	2	3	4	5	6	7	8	9	10

Notes: _____
_____
_____
_____

Overall score of the day

DAILY TRACKER

Date: _____

(M) (T) (W) (T) (F) (S) (S)

Menstrual cycle day _____

Breakfast
_____
_____

Lunch:
_____
_____

Dinner:
_____
_____

Supplements:
_____
_____

Medicines:
_____
_____

Pain Assessment

Pelvic	0	1	2	3	4	5	6	7	8	9	10
Abdominal	0	1	2	3	4	5	6	7	8	9	10
Rectal	0	1	2	3	4	5	6	7	8	9	10
Musculo skeletal	0	1	2	3	4	5	6	7	8	9	10
Sexual	0	1	2	3	4	5	6	7	8	9	10

Notes: _____
_____
_____
_____

Overall score of the day

DAILY TRACKER

Date: _____

(M) (T) (W) (T) (F) (S) (S)

Menstrual cycle day _____

Breakfast
_____
_____

Lunch:
_____
_____

Dinner:
_____
_____

Supplements:
_____
_____

Medicines:
_____
_____

Pain Assessment

| Pelvic | 0 | 1 | 2 | 3 | 4 | 5 | 6 | 7 | 8 | 9 | 10 |

| Abdominal | 0 | 1 | 2 | 3 | 4 | 5 | 6 | 7 | 8 | 9 | 10 |

| Rectal | 0 | 1 | 2 | 3 | 4 | 5 | 6 | 7 | 8 | 9 | 10 |

| Musculo skeletal | 0 | 1 | 2 | 3 | 4 | 5 | 6 | 7 | 8 | 9 | 10 |

| Sexual | 0 | 1 | 2 | 3 | 4 | 5 | 6 | 7 | 8 | 9 | 10 |

Notes: _____

Overall score of the day

DAILY TRACKER

Date: _____

(M) (T) (W) (T) (F) (S) (S)

Breakfast
_____
_____

Lunch:
_____
_____

Dinner:
_____
_____

Menstrual cycle day _____

Supplements: _____
_____

Medicines: _____
_____
_____

Pain Assessment

Pelvic	0	1	2	3	4	5	6	7	8	9	10
Abdominal	0	1	2	3	4	5	6	7	8	9	10
Rectal	0	1	2	3	4	5	6	7	8	9	10
Musculo skeletal	0	1	2	3	4	5	6	7	8	9	10
Sexual	0	1	2	3	4	5	6	7	8	9	10

Notes: _____
_____
_____
_____

Overall score of the day

DAILY TRACKER

Date: _____

Ⓜ Ⓣ Ⓦ Ⓣ Ⓕ Ⓢ Ⓢ

Menstrual cycle day _____

Breakfast

Supplements:

Lunch:

Dinner:

Medicines:

Pain Assessment

Pelvic	0	1	2	3	4	5	6	7	8	9	10
Abdominal	0	1	2	3	4	5	6	7	8	9	10
Rectal	0	1	2	3	4	5	6	7	8	9	10
Musculo skeletal	0	1	2	3	4	5	6	7	8	9	10
Sexual	0	1	2	3	4	5	6	7	8	9	10

Notes: _____

Overall score of the day

DAILY TRACKER

Date: _____

M T W T F S S

Menstrual cycle day _____

Breakfast
_____
_____

Lunch:
_____
_____

Dinner:
_____
_____

Supplements:
_____
_____

Medicines:
_____
_____

Pain Assessment

Pelvic | 0 | 1 | 2 | 3 | 4 | 5 | 6 | 7 | 8 | 9 | 10 |

Abdominal | 0 | 1 | 2 | 3 | 4 | 5 | 6 | 7 | 8 | 9 | 10 |

Rectal | 0 | 1 | 2 | 3 | 4 | 5 | 6 | 7 | 8 | 9 | 10 |

Musculo skeletal | 0 | 1 | 2 | 3 | 4 | 5 | 6 | 7 | 8 | 9 | 10 |

Sexual | 0 | 1 | 2 | 3 | 4 | 5 | 6 | 7 | 8 | 9 | 10 |

Notes: _____
_____
_____

Overall score of the day

DAILY TRACKER

Date: _____

M T W T F S S

Menstrual cycle day _____

Breakfast
_____
_____

Lunch:
_____
_____

Dinner:
_____
_____

Supplements:
_____
_____

Medicines:
_____
_____

Pain Assessment

Pelvic	0	1	2	3	4	5	6	7	8	9	10
Abdominal	0	1	2	3	4	5	6	7	8	9	10
Rectal	0	1	2	3	4	5	6	7	8	9	10
Musculo skeletal	0	1	2	3	4	5	6	7	8	9	10
Sexual	0	1	2	3	4	5	6	7	8	9	10

Notes: _____
_____
_____
_____

Overall score of the day

DAILY TRACKER

Date: _____

Ⓜ Ⓣ Ⓦ Ⓣ Ⓕ Ⓢ Ⓢ

Breakfast
_____
_____

Lunch:
_____
_____

Dinner:
_____
_____

Menstrual cycle day _____

Supplements:
_____
_____

Medicines:
_____
_____

Pain Assessment

Pelvic	0	1	2	3	4	5	6	7	8	9	10
Abdominal	0	1	2	3	4	5	6	7	8	9	10
Rectal	0	1	2	3	4	5	6	7	8	9	10
Musculo skeletal	0	1	2	3	4	5	6	7	8	9	10
Sexual	0	1	2	3	4	5	6	7	8	9	10

Notes: _____
_____
_____
_____

Overall score of the day

DAILY TRACKER

Date: _____

Ⓜ Ⓣ Ⓦ Ⓣ Ⓕ Ⓢ Ⓢ

Menstrual cycle day _____

Breakfast
_____
_____

Lunch:
_____
_____

Dinner:
_____
_____

Supplements:
_____
_____

Medicines:
_____
_____

Pain Assessment

Pelvic	0	1	2	3	4	5	6	7	8	9	10
Abdominal	0	1	2	3	4	5	6	7	8	9	10
Rectal	0	1	2	3	4	5	6	7	8	9	10
Musculo skeletal	0	1	2	3	4	5	6	7	8	9	10
Sexual	0	1	2	3	4	5	6	7	8	9	10

Notes: _____
_____
_____
_____

Overall score of the day

DAILY TRACKER

Date: _____

(M) (T) (W) (T) (F) (S) (S)

Menstrual cycle day _____

Breakfast
_____
_____

Lunch:
_____
_____

Dinner:
_____
_____

Supplements:
_____
_____

Medicines:
_____
_____

Pain Assessment

Pelvic	0	1	2	3	4	5	6	7	8	9	10
Abdominal	0	1	2	3	4	5	6	7	8	9	10
Rectal	0	1	2	3	4	5	6	7	8	9	10
Musculo skeletal	0	1	2	3	4	5	6	7	8	9	10
Sexual	0	1	2	3	4	5	6	7	8	9	10

Notes: _____
_____
_____

Overall score of the day

DAILY TRACKER

Date: _____

Ⓜ Ⓣ Ⓦ Ⓣ Ⓕ Ⓢ Ⓢ

Menstrual cycle day _____

Breakfast
_____
_____

Lunch:
_____
_____

Dinner:
_____
_____

Supplements:
_____
_____

Medicines:
_____
_____

Pain Assessment

Pelvic	0	1	2	3	4	5	6	7	8	9	10
Abdominal	0	1	2	3	4	5	6	7	8	9	10
Rectal	0	1	2	3	4	5	6	7	8	9	10
Musculo skeletal	0	1	2	3	4	5	6	7	8	9	10
Sexual	0	1	2	3	4	5	6	7	8	9	10

Notes: _____
_____
_____
_____

Overall score of the day

DAILY TRACKER

Date: _____

(M) (T) (W) (T) (F) (S) (S)

Menstrual cycle day _____

Breakfast
_____
_____

Supplements:
_____
_____

Lunch:
_____
_____

Medicines:
_____

Dinner:
_____
_____

Pain Assessment

Pelvic	0	1	2	3	4	5	6	7	8	9	10
Abdominal	0	1	2	3	4	5	6	7	8	9	10
Rectal	0	1	2	3	4	5	6	7	8	9	10
Musculo skeletal	0	1	2	3	4	5	6	7	8	9	10
Sexual	0	1	2	3	4	5	6	7	8	9	10

Notes: _____
_____
_____
_____

Overall score of the day

( )

DAILY TRACKER

Date: _____

Ⓜ Ⓣ Ⓦ Ⓣ Ⓕ Ⓢ Ⓢ

Menstrual cycle day _____

Breakfast
_____
_____

Lunch:
_____
_____

Dinner:
_____
_____

Supplements:
_____
_____
_____

Medicines:
_____
_____
_____

Pain Assessment

Pelvic	0	1	2	3	4	5	6	7	8	9	10
Abdominal	0	1	2	3	4	5	6	7	8	9	10
Rectal	0	1	2	3	4	5	6	7	8	9	10
Musculo skeletal	0	1	2	3	4	5	6	7	8	9	10
Sexual	0	1	2	3	4	5	6	7	8	9	10

Notes: _____
_____
_____
_____

Overall score of the day

◯

DAILY TRACKER

Date: _____

Ⓜ Ⓣ Ⓦ Ⓣ Ⓕ Ⓢ Ⓢ

Menstrual cycle day _____

Breakfast
_____
_____

Supplements:
_____
_____

Lunch:
_____
_____

Medicines:
_____
_____

Dinner:
_____
_____

Pain Assessment

Pelvic	0	1	2	3	4	5	6	7	8	9	10
Abdominal	0	1	2	3	4	5	6	7	8	9	10
Rectal	0	1	2	3	4	5	6	7	8	9	10
Musculo skeletal	0	1	2	3	4	5	6	7	8	9	10
Sexual	0	1	2	3	4	5	6	7	8	9	10

Notes: _____
_____
_____

Overall score of the day

DAILY TRACKER

Date: _____

Ⓜ Ⓣ Ⓦ Ⓣ Ⓕ Ⓢ Ⓢ

Menstrual cycle day _____

Breakfast
_____
_____

Supplements:
_____
_____

Lunch:
_____
_____

Medicines:
_____

Dinner:
_____
_____

_____

Pain Assessment

Pelvic	0	1	2	3	4	5	6	7	8	9	10
Abdominal	0	1	2	3	4	5	6	7	8	9	10
Rectal	0	1	2	3	4	5	6	7	8	9	10
Musculo skeletal	0	1	2	3	4	5	6	7	8	9	10
Sexual	0	1	2	3	4	5	6	7	8	9	10

Notes: _____
_____
_____
_____

Overall score of the day

( )

DAILY TRACKER

Date: _____

(M) (T) (W) (T) (F) (S) (S)

Breakfast
_____
_____

Lunch:
_____
_____

Dinner:
_____
_____

Menstrual cycle day _____

Supplements:
_____
_____

Medicines:
_____
_____

Pain Assessment

Pelvic	0	1	2	3	4	5	6	7	8	9	10
Abdominal	0	1	2	3	4	5	6	7	8	9	10
Rectal	0	1	2	3	4	5	6	7	8	9	10
Musculo skeletal	0	1	2	3	4	5	6	7	8	9	10
Sexual	0	1	2	3	4	5	6	7	8	9	10

Notes: _____
_____
_____
_____

Overall score of the day

( )

DAILY TRACKER

Date: _____

(M) (T) (W) (T) (F) (S) (S)

Menstrual cycle day _____

Breakfast
_____
_____

Lunch:
_____
_____

Dinner:
_____
_____

Supplements:
_____
_____
_____

Medicines:
_____
_____
_____

Pain Assessment

	0	1	2	3	4	5	6	7	8	9	10
Pelvic	0	1	2	3	4	5	6	7	8	9	10
Abdominal	0	1	2	3	4	5	6	7	8	9	10
Rectal	0	1	2	3	4	5	6	7	8	9	10
Musculo skeletal	0	1	2	3	4	5	6	7	8	9	10
Sexual	0	1	2	3	4	5	6	7	8	9	10

Notes: _____
_____
_____
_____

Overall score of the day

DAILY TRACKER

Date: _____

M T W T F S S

Menstrual
cycle day _____

Breakfast
_____
_____

Lunch:
_____
_____

Dinner:
_____
_____

Supplements:
_____
_____

Medicines:
_____
_____

Pain Assessment

Pelvic	0	1	2	3	4	5	6	7	8	9	10
Abdominal	0	1	2	3	4	5	6	7	8	9	10
Rectal	0	1	2	3	4	5	6	7	8	9	10
Musculo skeletal	0	1	2	3	4	5	6	7	8	9	10
Sexual	0	1	2	3	4	5	6	7	8	9	10

Notes: _____
_____
_____

Overall score of the day

DAILY TRACKER

Date: _____

Ⓜ Ⓣ Ⓦ Ⓣ Ⓕ Ⓢ Ⓢ

Menstrual cycle day _____

Breakfast
_____
_____

Supplements:
_____
_____

Lunch:
_____
_____

Medicines:
_____

Dinner:
_____
_____
_____

Pain Assessment

Pelvic	0	1	2	3	4	5	6	7	8	9	10
Abdominal	0	1	2	3	4	5	6	7	8	9	10
Rectal	0	1	2	3	4	5	6	7	8	9	10
Musculo skeletal	0	1	2	3	4	5	6	7	8	9	10
Sexual	0	1	2	3	4	5	6	7	8	9	10

Notes: _____
_____
_____
_____

Overall score of the day

DAILY TRACKER

Date: _____

(M) (T) (W) (T) (F) (S) (S)

Breakfast _____

Menstrual cycle day _____

_____

Supplements: _____

Lunch: _____

_____

_____

_____

Dinner: _____

Medicines: _____

_____

_____

Pain Assessment

Pelvic | 0 | 1 | 2 | 3 | 4 | 5 | 6 | 7 | 8 | 9 | 10 |

Abdominal | 0 | 1 | 2 | 3 | 4 | 5 | 6 | 7 | 8 | 9 | 10 |

Rectal | 0 | 1 | 2 | 3 | 4 | 5 | 6 | 7 | 8 | 9 | 10 |

Musculo skeletal | 0 | 1 | 2 | 3 | 4 | 5 | 6 | 7 | 8 | 9 | 10 |

Sexual | 0 | 1 | 2 | 3 | 4 | 5 | 6 | 7 | 8 | 9 | 10 |

Notes: _____

Overall score of the day

DAILY TRACKER

Date: _____

Ⓜ Ⓣ Ⓦ Ⓣ Ⓕ Ⓢ Ⓢ

Menstrual cycle day _____

Breakfast
_____
_____

Supplements:
_____
_____

Lunch:
_____
_____

Medicines:
_____
_____

Dinner:
_____
_____

Pain Assessment

Pelvic	0	1	2	3	4	5	6	7	8	9	10
Abdominal	0	1	2	3	4	5	6	7	8	9	10
Rectal	0	1	2	3	4	5	6	7	8	9	10
Musculo skeletal	0	1	2	3	4	5	6	7	8	9	10
Sexual	0	1	2	3	4	5	6	7	8	9	10

Notes: _____
_____
_____

Overall score of the day

DAILY TRACKER

Date: _____

M T W T F S S

Menstrual cycle day _____

Breakfast
_____
_____

Lunch:
_____
_____

Dinner:
_____
_____

Supplements:
_____
_____

Medicines:
_____
_____

Pain Assessment

Pelvic	0	1	2	3	4	5	6	7	8	9	10
Abdominal	0	1	2	3	4	5	6	7	8	9	10
Rectal	0	1	2	3	4	5	6	7	8	9	10
Musculo skeletal	0	1	2	3	4	5	6	7	8	9	10
Sexual	0	1	2	3	4	5	6	7	8	9	10

Notes: _____
_____
_____
_____

Overall score of the day

DAILY TRACKER

Date: _____

M T W T F S S

Menstrual cycle day _____

Breakfast
_____
_____

Lunch:
_____
_____

Dinner:
_____
_____

Supplements:
_____
_____

Medicines:
_____
_____

Pain Assessment

	0	1	2	3	4	5	6	7	8	9	10
Pelvic	0	1	2	3	4	5	6	7	8	9	10
Abdominal	0	1	2	3	4	5	6	7	8	9	10
Rectal	0	1	2	3	4	5	6	7	8	9	10
Musculo skeletal	0	1	2	3	4	5	6	7	8	9	10
Sexual	0	1	2	3	4	5	6	7	8	9	10

Notes: _____
_____
_____

Overall score of the day

DAILY TRACKER

Date: _____

Ⓜ Ⓣ Ⓦ Ⓣ Ⓕ Ⓢ Ⓢ

Menstrual cycle day _____

Breakfast
_____
_____

Supplements:
_____
_____

Lunch:
_____
_____

Dinner:
_____
_____

Medicines:
_____
_____

Pain Assessment

| Pelvic | 0 | 1 | 2 | 3 | 4 | 5 | 6 | 7 | 8 | 9 | 10 |

| Abdominal | 0 | 1 | 2 | 3 | 4 | 5 | 6 | 7 | 8 | 9 | 10 |

| Rectal | 0 | 1 | 2 | 3 | 4 | 5 | 6 | 7 | 8 | 9 | 10 |

| Musculo skeletal | 0 | 1 | 2 | 3 | 4 | 5 | 6 | 7 | 8 | 9 | 10 |

| Sexual | 0 | 1 | 2 | 3 | 4 | 5 | 6 | 7 | 8 | 9 | 10 |

Notes: _____
_____
_____
_____

Overall score of the day

DAILY TRACKER

Date: _____

(M) (T) (W) (T) (F) (S) (S)

Menstrual cycle day _____

Breakfast
_____
_____

Lunch:
_____
_____

Dinner:
_____
_____

Supplements:
_____
_____
_____

Medicines:
_____
_____
_____

Pain Assessment

| Pelvic | 0 | 1 | 2 | 3 | 4 | 5 | 6 | 7 | 8 | 9 | 10 |

| Abdominal | 0 | 1 | 2 | 3 | 4 | 5 | 6 | 7 | 8 | 9 | 10 |

| Rectal | 0 | 1 | 2 | 3 | 4 | 5 | 6 | 7 | 8 | 9 | 10 |

| Musculo skeletal | 0 | 1 | 2 | 3 | 4 | 5 | 6 | ·7 | 8 | 9 | 10 |

| Sexual | 0 | 1 | 2 | 3 | 4 | 5 | 6 | 7 | 8 | 9 | 10 |

Notes: _____
_____
_____

Overall score of the day

DAILY TRACKER

Date: _____

Ⓜ Ⓣ Ⓦ Ⓣ Ⓕ Ⓢ Ⓢ

Menstrual cycle day _____

Breakfast
_____
_____

Supplements:
_____
_____

Lunch:
_____
_____

Medicines:
_____

Dinner:
_____
_____
_____

Pain Assessment

Pelvic	0	1	2	3	4	5	6	7	8	9	10
Abdominal	0	1	2	3	4	5	6	7	8	9	10
Rectal	0	1	2	3	4	5	6	7	8	9	10
Musculo skeletal	0	1	2	3	4	5	6	7	8	9	10
Sexual	0	1	2	3	4	5	6	7	8	9	10

Notes: _____
_____
_____
_____

Overall score of the day

DAILY TRACKER

Date: _____

Ⓜ Ⓣ Ⓦ Ⓣ Ⓕ Ⓢ Ⓢ

Menstrual cycle day _____

Breakfast
_____
_____

Lunch:
_____
_____

Dinner:
_____
_____

Supplements:
_____
_____

Medicines:
_____
_____

Pain Assessment

	0	1	2	3	4	5	6	7	8	9	10
Pelvic	0	1	2	3	4	5	6	7	8	9	10
Abdominal	0	1	2	3	4	5	6	7	8	9	10
Rectal	0	1	2	3	4	5	6	7	8	9	10
Musculo skeletal	0	1	2	3	4	5	6	7	8	9	10
Sexual	0	1	2	3	4	5	6	7	8	9	10

Notes: _____
_____
_____
_____

Overall score of the day

DAILY TRACKER

Date: _____

M T W T F S S

Menstrual
cycle day _____

Breakfast
_____
_____

Supplements:
_____
_____

Lunch:
_____
_____

Medicines:
_____

Dinner:
_____
_____

Pain Assessment

| Pelvic | 0 | 1 | 2 | 3 | 4 | 5 | 6 | 7 | 8 | 9 | 10 |

| Abdominal | 0 | 1 | 2 | 3 | 4 | 5 | 6 | 7 | 8 | 9 | 10 |

| Rectal | 0 | 1 | 2 | 3 | 4 | 5 | 6 | 7 | 8 | 9 | 10 |

| Musculo skeletal | 0 | 1 | 2 | 3 | 4 | 5 | 6 | 7 | 8 | 9 | 10 |

| Sexual | 0 | 1 | 2 | 3 | 4 | 5 | 6 | 7 | 8 | 9 | 10 |

Notes: _____
_____
_____
_____

Overall score of the day

DAILY TRACKER

Date: _____

(M) (T) (W) (T) (F) (S) (S)

Menstrual cycle day _____

Breakfast
_____
_____

Lunch:
_____
_____

Dinner:
_____
_____

Supplements:
_____
_____
_____

Medicines:
_____
_____
_____

Pain Assessment

Pelvic	0	1	2	3	4	5	6	7	8	9	10
Abdominal	0	1	2	3	4	5	6	7	8	9	10
Rectal	0	1	2	3	4	5	6	7	8	9	10
Musculoskeletal	0	1	2	3	4	5	6	7	8	9	10
Sexual	0	1	2	3	4	5	6	7	8	9	10

Notes: _____
_____
_____
_____

Overall score of the day

DAILY TRACKER

Date: _____

Ⓜ Ⓣ Ⓦ Ⓣ Ⓕ Ⓢ Ⓢ

Menstrual cycle day _____

Breakfast
_____
_____

Supplements:
_____
_____

Lunch:
_____
_____

Dinner:
_____
_____

Medicines:
_____
_____

Pain Assessment

Pelvic	0	1	2	3	4	5	6	7	8	9	10
Abdominal	0	1	2	3	4	5	6	7	8	9	10
Rectal	0	1	2	3	4	5	6	7	8	9	10
Musculo skeletal	0	1	2	3	4	5	6	7	8	9	10
Sexual	0	1	2	3	4	5	6	7	8	9	10

Notes: _____
_____
_____
_____

Overall score of the day

DAILY TRACKER

Date: _____

Ⓜ Ⓣ Ⓦ Ⓣ Ⓕ Ⓢ Ⓢ

Menstrual cycle day _____

Breakfast
_____
_____

Lunch:
_____
_____

Dinner:
_____
_____

Supplements:
_____
_____

Medicines:
_____
_____

Pain Assessment

	0	1	2	3	4	5	6	7	8	9	10
Pelvic	0	1	2	3	4	5	6	7	8	9	10
Abdominal	0	1	2	3	4	5	6	7	8	9	10
Rectal	0	1	2	3	4	5	6	7	8	9	10
Musculo skeletal	0	1	2	3	4	5	6	7	8	9	10
Sexual	0	1	2	3	4	5	6	7	8	9	10

Notes: _____
_____
_____
_____

Overall score of the day

DAILY TRACKER

Date: _____

Ⓜ Ⓣ Ⓦ Ⓣ Ⓕ Ⓢ Ⓢ

Menstrual
cycle day _____

Breakfast
_____
_____

Supplements:
_____
_____

Lunch:
_____
_____

Medicines:
_____

Dinner:
_____
_____

Pain Assessment

Pelvic	0	1	2	3	4	5	6	7	8	9	10

Abdominal	0	1	2	3	4	5	6	7	8	9	10

Rectal	0	1	2	3	4	5	6	7	8	9	10

Musculo skeletal	0	1	2	3	4	5	6	7	8	9	10

Sexual	0	1	2	3	4	5	6	7	8	9	10

Notes: _____
_____
_____
_____

Overall score of the day

DAILY TRACKER

Date: _____

M T W T F S S

Menstrual
cycle day _____

Breakfast
_____
_____

Lunch:
_____
_____

Dinner:
_____
_____

Supplements:
_____
_____

Medicines:
_____
_____

Pain Assessment

Pelvic	0	1	2	3	4	5	6	7	8	9	10
Abdominal	0	1	2	3	4	5	6	7	8	9	10
Rectal	0	1	2	3	4	5	6	7	8	9	10
Musculo skeletal	0	1	2	3	4	5	6	7	8	9	10
Sexual	0	1	2	3	4	5	6	7	8	9	10

Notes: _____
_____
_____
_____

Overall score of the day

DAILY TRACKER

Date: _____

M T W T F S S

Menstrual cycle day _____

Breakfast
_____

_____

Lunch:
_____

_____

Dinner:
_____

_____

Supplements:
_____

_____

_____

Medicines:
_____

_____

_____

Pain Assessment

Pelvic	0	1	2	3	4	5	6	7	8	9	10
Abdominal	0	1	2	3	4	5	6	7	8	9	10
Rectal	0	1	2	3	4	5	6	7	8	9	10
Musculo skeletal	0	1	2	3	4	5	6	7	8	9	10
Sexual	0	1	2	3	4	5	6	7	8	9	10

Notes: _____

_____

_____

Overall score of the day

DAILY TRACKER

Date: _____

(M) (T) (W) (T) (F) (S) (S)

Menstrual cycle day _____

Breakfast
_____
_____

Lunch:
_____
_____

Dinner:
_____
_____

Supplements:
_____
_____

Medicines:
_____
_____

Pain Assessment

	0	1	2	3	4	5	6	7	8	9	10
Pelvic	0	1	2	3	4	5	6	7	8	9	10
Abdominal	0	1	2	3	4	5	6	7	8	9	10
Rectal	0	1	2	3	4	5	6	7	8	9	10
Musculo skeletal	0	1	2	3	4	5	6	7	8	9	10
Sexual	0	1	2	3	4	5	6	7	8	9	10

Notes: _____
_____
_____
_____

Overall score of the day

DAILY TRACKER

Date: _____

Ⓜ Ⓣ Ⓦ Ⓣ Ⓕ Ⓢ Ⓢ

Menstrual cycle day _____

Breakfast
_____
_____

Supplements:
_____
_____

Lunch:
_____
_____

Medicines:
_____

Dinner:
_____
_____
_____

Pain Assessment

Pelvic	0	1	2	3	4	5	6	7	8	9	10
Abdominal	0	1	2	3	4	5	6	7	8	9	10
Rectal	0	1	2	3	4	5	6	7	8	9	10
Musculo skeletal	0	1	2	3	4	5	6	7	8	9	10
Sexual	0	1	2	3	4	5	6	7	8	9	10

Notes: _____
_____
_____
_____

Overall score of the day

DAILY TRACKER

Date: _____

(M) (T) (W) (T) (F) (S) (S)

Menstrual cycle day _____

Breakfast
_____
_____

Lunch:
_____
_____

Dinner:
_____
_____

Supplements:
_____
_____
_____

Medicines:
_____
_____
_____

Pain Assessment

Pelvic	0	1	2	3	4	5	6	7	8	9	10
Abdominal	0	1	2	3	4	5	6	7	8	9	10
Rectal	0	1	2	3	4	5	6	7	8	9	10
Musculo skeletal	0	1	2	3	4	5	6	7	8	9	10
Sexual	0	1	2	3	4	5	6	7	8	9	10

Notes: _____
_____
_____
_____

Overall score of the day

DAILY TRACKER

Date: _____

Ⓜ Ⓣ Ⓦ Ⓣ Ⓕ Ⓢ Ⓢ

Menstrual cycle day _____

Breakfast
_____
_____

Lunch:
_____
_____

Dinner:
_____
_____

Supplements:
_____
_____

Medicines:
_____
_____

Pain Assessment

Pelvic	0	1	2	3	4	5	6	7	8	9	10
Abdominal	0	1	2	3	4	5	6	7	8	9	10
Rectal	0	1	2	3	4	5	6	7	8	9	10
Musculo skeletal	0	1	2	3	4	5	6	7	8	9	10
Sexual	0	1	2	3	4	5	6	7	8	9	10

Notes: _____
_____
_____

Overall score of the day

DAILY TRACKER

Date: _____

Ⓜ Ⓣ Ⓦ Ⓣ Ⓕ Ⓢ Ⓢ

Menstrual cycle day _____

Breakfast
_____
_____

Lunch:
_____
_____

Dinner:
_____
_____

Supplements:
_____
_____

Medicines:
_____
_____

Pain Assessment

	0	1	2	3	4	5	6	7	8	9	10
Pelvic	0	1	2	3	4	5	6	7	8	9	10
Abdominal	0	1	2	3	4	5	6	7	8	9	10
Rectal	0	1	2	3	4	5	6	7	8	9	10
Musculo skeletal	0	1	2	3	4	5	6	7	8	9	10
Sexual	0	1	2	3	4	5	6	7	8	9	10

Notes: _____
_____
_____
_____

Overall score of the day

DAILY TRACKER

Date: _____

M T W T F S S

Menstrual cycle day _____

Breakfast
_____
_____

Lunch:
_____
_____

Dinner:
_____
_____

Supplements:
_____
_____

Medicines:
_____
_____

Pain Assessment

| Pelvic | 0 | 1 | 2 | 3 | 4 | 5 | 6 | 7 | 8 | 9 | 10 |

| Abdominal | 0 | 1 | 2 | 3 | 4 | 5 | 6 | 7 | 8 | 9 | 10 |

| Rectal | 0 | 1 | 2 | 3 | 4 | 5 | 6 | 7 | 8 | 9 | 10 |

| Musculo skeletal | 0 | 1 | 2 | 3 | 4 | 5 | 6 | 7 | 8 | 9 | 10 |

| Sexual | 0 | 1 | 2 | 3 | 4 | 5 | 6 | 7 | 8 | 9 | 10 |

Notes: _____
_____
_____
_____

Overall score of the day

DAILY TRACKER

Date: _____

Ⓜ Ⓣ Ⓦ Ⓣ Ⓕ Ⓢ Ⓢ

Menstrual cycle day _____

Breakfast
_____
_____

Lunch:
_____
_____

Dinner:
_____
_____

Supplements:
_____
_____

Medicines:
_____
_____

Pain Assessment

Pelvic	0	1	2	3	4	5	6	7	8	9	10
Abdominal	0	1	2	3	4	5	6	7	8	9	10
Rectal	0	1	2	3	4	5	6	7	8	9	10
Musculo skeletal	0	1	2	3	4	5	6	7	8	9	10
Sexual	0	1	2	3	4	5	6	7	8	9	10

Notes: _____
_____
_____
_____

Overall score of the day

DAILY TRACKER

Date: _____

Ⓜ Ⓣ Ⓦ Ⓣ Ⓕ Ⓢ Ⓢ

Menstrual cycle day _____

Breakfast
_____
_____

Supplements:
_____
_____

Lunch:
_____
_____

Medicines:
_____

Dinner:
_____
_____

Pain Assessment

| Pelvic | 0 | 1 | 2 | 3 | 4 | 5 | 6 | 7 | 8 | 9 | 10 |

| Abdominal | 0 | 1 | 2 | 3 | 4 | 5 | 6 | 7 | 8 | 9 | 10 |

| Rectal | 0 | 1 | 2 | 3 | 4 | 5 | 6 | 7 | 8 | 9 | 10 |

| Musculo skeletal | 0 | 1 | 2 | 3 | 4 | 5 | 6 | 7 | 8 | 9 | 10 |

| Sexual | 0 | 1 | 2 | 3 | 4 | 5 | 6 | 7 | 8 | 9 | 10 |

Notes: _____
_____
_____

Overall score of the day
◯

DAILY TRACKER

Date: _____

(M) (T) (W) (T) (F) (S) (S)

Breakfast
_____
_____

Lunch:
_____
_____

Dinner:
_____
_____

Menstrual cycle day _____

Supplements:
_____
_____

Medicines:
_____
_____

Pain Assessment

Pelvic	0	1	2	3	4	5	6	7	8	9	10
Abdominal	0	1	2	3	4	5	6	7	8	9	10
Rectal	0	1	2	3	4	5	6	7	8	9	10
Musculo skeletal	0	1	2	3	4	5	6	7	8	9	10
Sexual	0	1	2	3	4	5	6	7	8	9	10

Notes: _____
_____
_____
_____

Overall score of the day

DAILY TRACKER

Date: _____

(M) (T) (W) (T) (F) (S) (S)

Menstrual cycle day _____

Breakfast
_____
_____

Lunch:
_____
_____

Dinner:
_____
_____

Supplements:
_____
_____

Medicines:
_____
_____

Pain Assessment

Pelvic | 0 | 1 | 2 | 3 | 4 | 5 | 6 | 7 | 8 | 9 | 10 |

Abdominal | 0 | 1 | 2 | 3 | 4 | 5 | 6 | 7 | 8 | 9 | 10 |

Rectal | 0 | 1 | 2 | 3 | 4 | 5 | 6 | 7 | 8 | 9 | 10 |

Musculo skeletal | 0 | 1 | 2 | 3 | 4 | 5 | 6 | 7 | 8 | 9 | 10 |

Sexual | 0 | 1 | 2 | 3 | 4 | 5 | 6 | 7 | 8 | 9 | 10 |

Notes: _____
_____
_____

Overall score of the day

DAILY TRACKER

Date: _____

(M) (T) (W) (T) (F) (S) (S)

Breakfast _____

Menstrual cycle day _____

Supplements: _____

Lunch: _____

Dinner: _____

Medicines: _____

Pain Assessment

	0	1	2	3	4	5	6	7	8	9	10
Pelvic	0	1	2	3	4	5	6	7	8	9	10
Abdominal	0	1	2	3	4	5	6	7	8	9	10
Rectal	0	1	2	3	4	5	6	7	8	9	10
Musculoskeletal	0	1	2	3	4	5	6	7	8	9	10
Sexual	0	1	2	3	4	5	6	7	8	9	10

Notes: _____

Overall score of the day

DAILY TRACKER

Date: _____

Ⓜ Ⓣ Ⓦ Ⓣ Ⓕ Ⓢ Ⓢ

Menstrual cycle day _____

Breakfast
_____
_____

Supplements:
_____
_____

Lunch:
_____
_____

Medicines:
_____

Dinner:
_____
_____

Pain Assessment

Pelvic	0	1	2	3	4	5	6	7	8	9	10
Abdominal	0	1	2	3	4	5	6	7	8	9	10
Rectal	0	1	2	3	4	5	6	7	8	9	10
Musculo skeletal	0	1	2	3	4	5	6	7	8	9	10
Sexual	0	1	2	3	4	5	6	7	8	9	10

Notes: _____
_____
_____
_____

Overall score of the day

DAILY TRACKER

Date: _____

Ⓜ Ⓣ Ⓦ Ⓣ Ⓕ Ⓢ Ⓢ

Menstrual cycle day _____

Breakfast
_____
_____

Lunch:
_____
_____

Dinner:
_____
_____

Supplements:
_____
_____

Medicines:
_____
_____

Pain Assessment

	0	1	2	3	4	5	6	7	8	9	10
Pelvic	0	1	2	3	4	5	6	7	8	9	10
Abdominal	0	1	2	3	4	5	6	7	8	9	10
Rectal	0	1	2	3	4	5	6	7	8	9	10
Musculo skeletal	0	1	2	3	4	5	6	7	8	9	10
Sexual	0	1	2	3	4	5	6	7	8	9	10

Notes: _____
_____
_____
_____

Overall score of the day

DAILY TRACKER

Date: _____

M T W T F S S

Menstrual cycle day _____

Breakfast
_____
_____

Lunch:
_____
_____

Dinner:
_____
_____

Supplements:
_____
_____
_____

Medicines:
_____
_____
_____

Pain Assessment

Pelvic	0	1	2	3	4	5	6	7	8	9	10
Abdominal	0	1	2	3	4	5	6	7	8	9	10
Rectal	0	1	2	3	4	5	6	7	8	9	10
Musculo skeletal	0	1	2	3	4	5	6	7	8	9	10
Sexual	0	1	2	3	4	5	6	7	8	9	10

Notes: _____
_____
_____

Overall score of the day

DAILY TRACKER

Date: _____

(M) (T) (W) (T) (F) (S) (S)

Breakfast _____
_____

Menstrual cycle day _____

Supplements: _____
_____

Lunch: _____
_____

Dinner: _____
_____

Medicines: _____
_____

Pain Assessment

Pelvic	0	1	2	3	4	5	6	7	8	9	10
Abdominal	0	1	2	3	4	5	6	7	8	9	10
Rectal	0	1	2	3	4	5	6	7	8	9	10
Musculo skeletal	0	1	2	3	4	5	6	7	8	9	10
Sexual	0	1	2	3	4	5	6	7	8	9	10

Notes: _____
_____
_____
_____

Overall score of the day

DAILY TRACKER

Date: _____

(M) (T) (W) (T) (F) (S) (S)

Menstrual cycle day _____

Breakfast
_____
_____

Lunch:
_____
_____

Dinner:
_____
_____

Supplements:
_____
_____

Medicines:
_____
_____

Pain Assessment

	0	1	2	3	4	5	6	7	8	9	10
Pelvic	0	1	2	3	4	5	6	7	8	9	10
Abdominal	0	1	2	3	4	5	6	7	8	9	10
Rectal	0	1	2	3	4	5	6	7	8	9	10
Musculo skeletal	0	1	2	3	4	5	6	7	8	9	10
Sexual	0	1	2	3	4	5	6	7	8	9	10

Notes: _____
_____
_____
_____

Overall score of the day

DAILY TRACKER

Date: _____

(M) (T) (W) (T) (F) (S) (S)

Menstrual cycle day _____

Breakfast
_____
_____

Lunch:
_____
_____

Dinner:
_____
_____

Supplements:
_____
_____

Medicines:
_____
_____
_____

Pain Assessment

	0	1	2	3	4	5	6	7	8	9	10
Pelvic	0	1	2	3	4	5	6	7	8	9	10
Abdominal	0	1	2	3	4	5	6	7	8	9	10
Rectal	0	1	2	3	4	5	6	7	8	9	10
Musculo skeletal	0	1	2	3	4	5	6	7	8	9	10
Sexual	0	1	2	3	4	5	6	7	8	9	10

Notes: _____
_____
_____
_____

Overall score of the day

DAILY TRACKER

Date: _____

M T W T F S S

Menstrual cycle day _____

Breakfast
_____
_____

Lunch:
_____
_____

Dinner:
_____
_____

Supplements:
_____
_____

Medicines:
_____
_____

Pain Assessment

Pelvic | 0 | 1 | 2 | 3 | 4 | 5 | 6 | 7 | 8 | 9 | 10

Abdominal | 0 | 1 | 2 | 3 | 4 | 5 | 6 | 7 | 8 | 9 | 10

Rectal | 0 | 1 | 2 | 3 | 4 | 5 | 6 | 7 | 8 | 9 | 10

Musculo skeletal | 0 | 1 | 2 | 3 | 4 | 5 | 6 | 7 | 8 | 9 | 10

Sexual | 0 | 1 | 2 | 3 | 4 | 5 | 6 | 7 | 8 | 9 | 10

Notes: _____
_____
_____

Overall score of the day

DAILY TRACKER

Date: _____

Ⓜ Ⓣ Ⓦ Ⓣ Ⓕ Ⓢ Ⓢ

Menstrual cycle day _____

Breakfast
_____
_____

Lunch:
_____
_____

Dinner:
_____
_____

Supplements:
_____
_____

Medicines:
_____
_____

Pain Assessment

Pelvic	0	1	2	3	4	5	6	7	8	9	10
Abdominal	0	1	2	3	4	5	6	7	8	9	10
Rectal	0	1	2	3	4	5	6	7	8	9	10
Musculo skeletal	0	1	2	3	4	5	6	7	8	9	10
Sexual	0	1	2	3	4	5	6	7	8	9	10

Notes: _____
_____
_____
_____

Overall score of the day

DAILY TRACKER

Date: _____

(M) (T) (W) (T) (F) (S) (S)

Menstrual cycle day _____

Breakfast
_____
_____

Supplements:
_____
_____

Lunch:
_____
_____

Medicines:
_____

Dinner:
_____
_____

Pain Assessment

Pelvic | 0 | 1 | 2 | 3 | 4 | 5 | 6 | 7 | 8 | 9 | 10 |

Abdominal | 0 | 1 | 2 | 3 | 4 | 5 | 6 | 7 | 8 | 9 | 10 |

Rectal | 0 | 1 | 2 | 3 | 4 | 5 | 6 | 7 | 8 | 9 | 10 |

Musculo skeletal | 0 | 1 | 2 | 3 | 4 | 5 | 6 | 7 | 8 | 9 | 10 |

Sexual | 0 | 1 | 2 | 3 | 4 | 5 | 6 | 7 | 8 | 9 | 10 |

Notes: _____
_____
_____

Overall score of the day

( )

DAILY TRACKER

Date: _____

(M) (T) (W) (T) (F) (S) (S)

Menstrual cycle day _____

Breakfast
_____
_____

Lunch:
_____
_____

Dinner:
_____
_____

Supplements:
_____
_____

Medicines:
_____
_____

Pain Assessment

Pelvic	0	1	2	3	4	5	6	7	8	9	10
Abdominal	0	1	2	3	4	5	6	7	8	9	10
Rectal	0	1	2	3	4	5	6	7	8	9	10
Musculo skeletal	0	1	2	3	4	5	6	7	8	9	10
Sexual	0	1	2	3	4	5	6	7	8	9	10

Notes: _____
_____
_____
_____

Overall score of the day

DAILY TRACKER

Date: _____

Ⓜ Ⓣ Ⓦ Ⓣ Ⓕ Ⓢ Ⓢ

Menstrual cycle day _____

Breakfast
....
....

Lunch:
....
....

Dinner:
....
....

Supplements:
....
....

Medicines:
....
....

Pain Assessment

Pelvic	0	1	2	3	4	5	6	7	8	9	10
Abdominal	0	1	2	3	4	5	6	7	8	9	10
Rectal	0	1	2	3	4	5	6	7	8	9	10
Musculo skeletal	0	1	2	3	4	5	6	7	8	9	10
Sexual	0	1	2	3	4	5	6	7	8	9	10

Notes: ....
....
....
....

Overall score of the day

DAILY TRACKER

Date: _____

(M) (T) (W) (T) (F) (S) (S)

Breakfast
_____
_____

Lunch:
_____
_____

Dinner:
_____
_____

Menstrual cycle day _____

Supplements:
_____
_____

Medicines:
_____
_____

Pain Assessment

Pelvic	0	1	2	3	4	5	6	7	8	9	10
Abdominal	0	1	2	3	4	5	6	7	8	9	10
Rectal	0	1	2	3	4	5	6	7	8	9	10
Musculo skeletal	0	1	2	3	4	5	6	7	8	9	10
Sexual	0	1	2	3	4	5	6	7	8	9	10

Notes: _____
_____
_____
_____

Overall score of the day

DAILY TRACKER

Date: _____

Ⓜ Ⓣ Ⓦ Ⓣ Ⓕ Ⓢ Ⓢ

Menstrual
cycle day _____

Breakfast
_____
_____

Supplements:
_____
_____

Lunch:
_____
_____

Medicines:
_____

Dinner:
_____
_____
_____

Pain Assessment

| Pelvic | 0 | 1 | 2 | 3 | 4 | 5 | 6 | 7 | 8 | 9 | 10 |

| Abdominal | 0 | 1 | 2 | 3 | 4 | 5 | 6 | 7 | 8 | 9 | 10 |

| Rectal | 0 | 1 | 2 | 3 | 4 | 5 | 6 | 7 | 8 | 9 | 10 |

| Musculo skeletal | 0 | 1 | 2 | 3 | 4 | 5 | 6 | 7 | 8 | 9 | 10 |

| Sexual | 0 | 1 | 2 | 3 | 4 | 5 | 6 | 7 | 8 | 9 | 10 |

Notes: _____
_____
_____

Overall score of the day

◯

DAILY TRACKER

Date: _____

M T W T F S S

Menstrual cycle day _____

Breakfast
_____
_____

Lunch:
_____
_____

Dinner:
_____
_____

Supplements:
_____
_____

Medicines:
_____
_____

Pain Assessment

| Pelvic | 0 | 1 | 2 | 3 | 4 | 5 | 6 | 7 | 8 | 9 | 10 |

| Abdominal | 0 | 1 | 2 | 3 | 4 | 5 | 6 | 7 | 8 | 9 | 10 |

| Rectal | 0 | 1 | 2 | 3 | 4 | 5 | 6 | 7 | 8 | 9 | 10 |

| Musculo skeletal | 0 | 1 | 2 | 3 | 4 | 5 | 6 | 7 | 8 | 9 | 10 |

| Sexual | 0 | 1 | 2 | 3 | 4 | 5 | 6 | 7 | 8 | 9 | 10 |

Notes: _____
_____
_____
_____

Overall score of the day

DAILY TRACKER

Date: _____

Ⓜ Ⓣ Ⓦ Ⓣ Ⓕ Ⓢ Ⓢ

Menstrual cycle day _____

Breakfast
_____
_____

Supplements:
_____
_____

Lunch:
_____
_____

Medicines:
_____

Dinner:
_____
_____

Pain Assessment

Pelvic	0	1	2	3	4	5	6	7	8	9	10
Abdominal	0	1	2	3	4	5	6	7	8	9	10
Rectal	0	1	2	3	4	5	6	7	8	9	10
Musculo skeletal	0	1	2	3	4	5	6	7	8	9	10
Sexual	0	1	2	3	4	5	6	7	8	9	10

Notes: _____
_____
_____
_____

Overall score of the day

◯

DAILY TRACKER

Date: _____

(M) (T) (W) (T) (F) (S) (S)

Menstrual cycle day _____

Breakfast
_____
_____

Lunch:
_____
_____

Dinner:
_____
_____

Supplements:
_____
_____

Medicines:
_____
_____

Pain Assessment

Pelvic	0	1	2	3	4	5	6	7	8	9	10
Abdominal	0	1	2	3	4	5	6	7	8	9	10
Rectal	0	1	2	3	4	5	6	7	8	9	10
Musculo skeletal	0	1	2	3	4	5	6	7	8	9	10
Sexual	0	1	2	3	4	5	6	7	8	9	10

Notes: _____
_____
_____
_____

Overall score of the day

◯

DAILY TRACKER

Date: _____

(M) (T) (W) (T) (F) (S) (S)

Menstrual cycle day _____

Breakfast
_____
_____

Supplements:
_____
_____

Lunch:
_____
_____

Medicines:
_____

Dinner:
_____
_____

Pain Assessment

Pelvic	0	1	2	3	4	5	6	7	8	9	10
Abdominal	0	1	2	3	4	5	6	7	8	9	10
Rectal	0	1	2	3	4	5	6	7	8	9	10
Musculo skeletal	0	1	2	3	4	5	6	7	8	9	10
Sexual	0	1	2	3	4	5	6	7	8	9	10

Notes: _____
_____
_____
_____

Overall score of the day

DAILY TRACKER

Date: _____

(M) (T) (W) (T) (F) (S) (S)

Breakfast
_____
_____

Lunch:
_____
_____

Dinner:
_____
_____

Menstrual cycle day _____

Supplements:
_____
_____

Medicines:
_____
_____

Pain Assessment

Pelvic	0	1	2	3	4	5	6	7	8	9	10
Abdominal	0	1	2	3	4	5	6	7	8	9	10
Rectal	0	1	2	3	4	5	6	7	8	9	10
Musculo skeletal	0	1	2	3	4	5	6	7	8	9	10
Sexual	0	1	2	3	4	5	6	7	8	9	10

Notes: _____
_____
_____
_____

Overall score of the day

DAILY TRACKER

Date: _____

Ⓜ Ⓣ Ⓦ Ⓣ Ⓕ Ⓢ Ⓢ

Menstrual cycle day _____

Breakfast
_____
_____

Supplements:
_____
_____

Lunch:
_____
_____

Medicines:
_____
_____

Dinner:
_____
_____

Pain Assessment

	0	1	2	3	4	5	6	7	8	9	10
Pelvic	0	1	2	3	4	5	6	7	8	9	10
Abdominal	0	1	2	3	4	5	6	7	8	9	10
Rectal	0	1	2	3	4	5	6	7	8	9	10
Musculo skeletal	0	1	2	3	4	5	6	7	8	9	10
Sexual	0	1	2	3	4	5	6	7	8	9	10

Notes: _____
_____
_____

Overall score of the day

DAILY TRACKER

Date: _____

Ⓜ Ⓣ Ⓦ Ⓣ Ⓕ Ⓢ Ⓢ

Menstrual cycle day _____

Breakfast
_____
_____

Lunch:
_____
_____

Dinner:
_____
_____

Supplements:
_____
_____

Medicines:
_____
_____

Pain Assessment

	0	1	2	3	4	5	6	7	8	9	10
Pelvic	0	1	2	3	4	5	6	7	8	9	10
Abdominal	0	1	2	3	4	5	6	7	8	9	10
Rectal	0	1	2	3	4	5	6	7	8	9	10
Musculo skeletal	0	1	2	3	4	5	6	7	8	9	10
Sexual	0	1	2	3	4	5	6	7	8	9	10

Notes: _____
_____
_____
_____

Overall score of the day

DAILY TRACKER

Breakfast
_____
_____

Lunch:
_____
_____

Dinner:
_____
_____

Date: _____

Ⓜ Ⓣ Ⓦ Ⓣ Ⓕ Ⓢ Ⓢ

Menstrual
cycle day _____

Supplements:
_____
_____

Medicines:
_____
_____

Pain Assessment

Pelvic	0	1	2	3	4	5	6	7	8	9	10
Abdominal	0	1	2	3	4	5	6	7	8	9	10
Rectal	0	1	2	3	4	5	6	7	8	9	10
Musculo skeletal	0	1	2	3	4	5	6	7	8	9	10
Sexual	0	1	2	3	4	5	6	7	8	9	10

Notes: _____
_____
_____
_____

Overall score of the day

Pain Level Trends

--> Add the overall score for every day you have recorded in your log sheets and plot a graph or colour the bar chart to create a trend graph for 30-day table.

--> Try to spot common patterns of food intake for days with high pain scores.

Date	0	1	2	3	4	5	6	7	8	9	10

Date	0	1	2	3	4	5	6	7	8	9	10

Date	0	1	2	3	4	5	6	7	8	9	10

Date	0	1	2	3	4	5	6	7	8	9	10

Date	0	1	2	3	4	5	6	7	8	9	10

Date	0	1	2	3	4	5	6	7	8	9	10

My Favourite Recipes

--> *Write down the recipes which you have found to be more compliant with your endometriosis condition and that you like the most.*

MY RECIPES

RECIPE: _____

INGREDIENTS **QUANTITY**

_____   _____
_____   _____
_____   _____
_____   _____
_____   _____
_____   _____

EXECUTION

_____
_____
_____
_____
_____
_____
_____
_____
_____
_____
_____
_____

MY RECIPES

RECIPE: ....

INGREDIENTS **QUANTITY**

EXECUTION

MY RECIPES

RECIPE: _____

INGREDIENTS	QUANTITY

EXECUTION

MY RECIPES

RECIPE: _____

INGREDIENTS　　　　　　　　　　　　　　　**QUANTITY**

_____　　_____
_____　　_____
_____　　_____
_____　　_____
_____　　_____
_____　　_____

EXECUTION

_____
_____
_____
_____
_____
_____
_____
_____
_____
_____
_____
_____

MY RECIPES

RECIPE: _____

INGREDIENTS　　　　　　　　　　　　　　　　**QUANTITY**

_____　　_____
_____　　_____
_____　　_____
_____　　_____
_____　　_____
_____　　_____

EXECUTION

_____
_____
_____
_____
_____
_____
_____
_____
_____
_____
_____
_____

MY RECIPES

RECIPE:

INGREDIENTS   QUANTITY

EXECUTION

MY RECIPES

RECIPE: _____

INGREDIENTS **QUANTITY**

_____ _____
_____ _____
_____ _____
_____ _____
_____ _____
_____ _____

EXECUTION

_____
_____
_____
_____
_____
_____
_____
_____
_____
_____
_____
_____

MY RECIPES

RECIPE:

INGREDIENTS **QUANTITY**

EXECUTION

MY RECIPES

RECIPE:

INGREDIENTS **QUANTITY**

EXECUTION

MY RECIPES

RECIPE: ....

INGREDIENTS　　　　　　　　　　　　　**QUANTITY**

EXECUTION

New series: 3 endometriosis journals from the same author

- Set of 90 daily tracking sheets, covering three months
- Daily tracker layout on two page spread allowing more space for journaling
- Endo girl profile cover

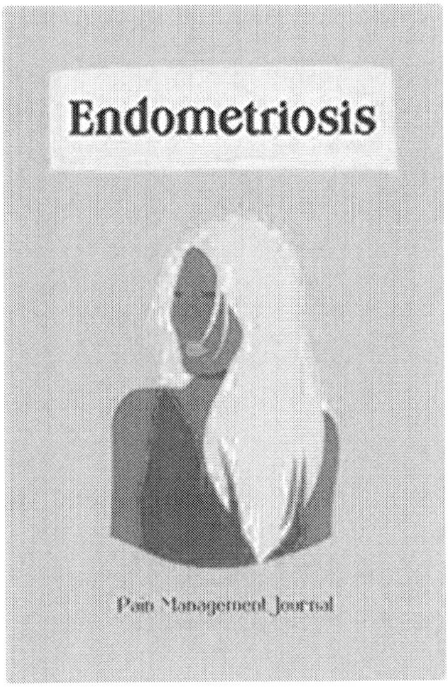
Endometriosis
Pain Management Journal

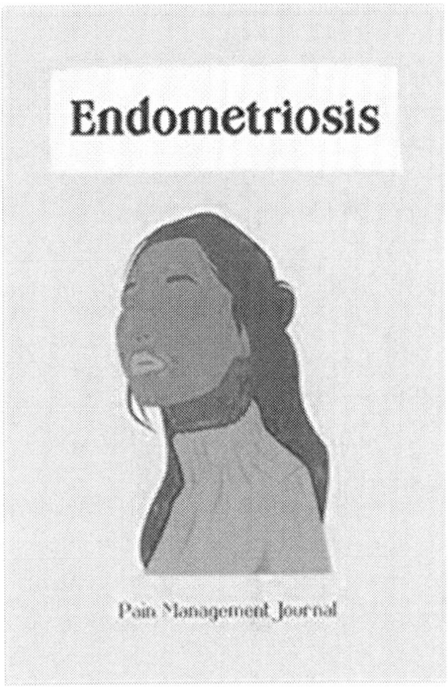
Endometriosis
Pain Management Journal

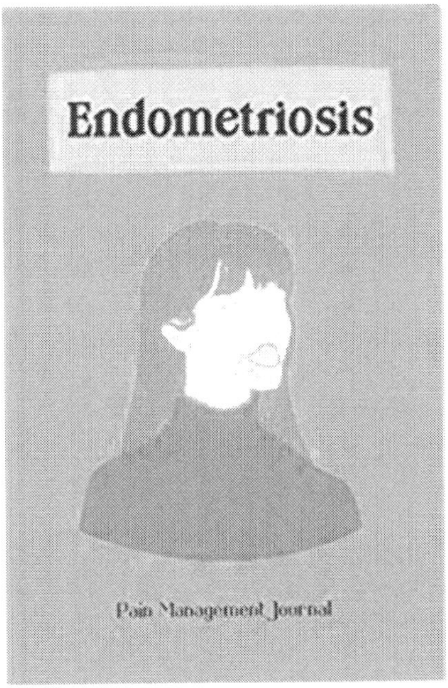
Endometriosis
Pain Management Journal

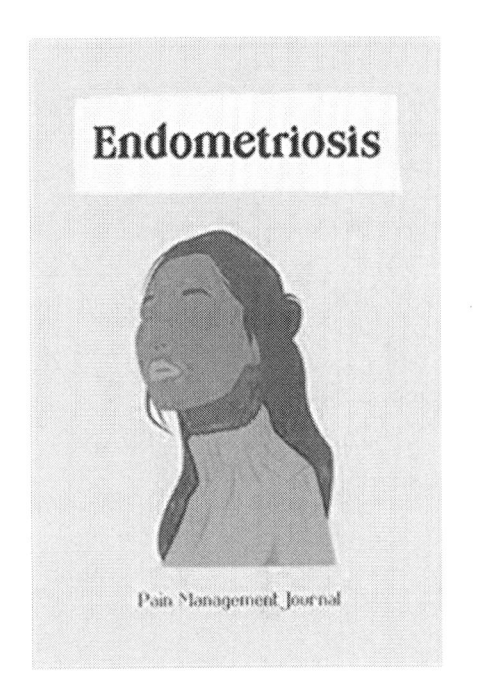

References

1. Zhang Y, Cao H, Yu Z, Peng HY, Zhang CJ. Curcumin inhibits endometriosis endometrial cells by reducing estradiol production. Iran J Reprod Med. 2013 May;11(5):415-22. PMID: 24639774; PMCID: PMC3941414.

2. Vallée A, Lecarpentier Y. Curcumin and Endometriosis. Int J Mol Sci. 2020 Mar 31;21(7):2440. doi: 10.3390/ijms21072440. PMID: 32244563; PMCID: PMC7177778.

3. Thomson CA, Ho E, Strom MB. Chemopreventive properties of 3,3'-diindolylmethane in breast cancer: evidence from experimental and human studies. Nutr Rev. 2016 Jul;74(7):432-43. doi: 10.1093/nutrit/nuw010. Epub 2016 May 31. PMID: 27261275; PMCID: PMC5059820.

4. Harris HR, Eke AC, Chavarro JE, Missmer SA. Fruit and vegetable consumption and risk of endometriosis. Hum Reprod. 2018 Apr 1;33(4):715-727. DOI: 10.1093/humrep/dey014. PMID: 29401293; PMCID: PMC6018917.

5. Parazzini F, Chiaffarino F, Surace M, Chatenoud L, Cipriani S, Chiantera V, Benzi G, Fedele L. Selected food intake and risk of endometriosis. Hum Reprod. 2004 Aug;19(8):1755-9. doi: 10.1093/humrep/deh395. Epub 2004 Jul 14. PMID: 15254009.

6. Gaskins AJ, Mumford SL, Zhang C, Wactawski-Wende J, Hovey KM, Whitcomb BW, Howards PP, Perkins NJ, Yeung E, Schisterman EF; BioCycle Study Group. Effect of daily fiber intake on reproductive function: the BioCycle Study. Am J Clin Nutr. 2009 Oct;90(4):1061-9. doi: 10.3945/ajcn.2009.27990. Epub 2009 Aug 19. PMID: 19692496; PMCID: PMC2744625.

7. Signorile PG, Viceconte R, Baldi A. Novel dietary supplement association reduces symptoms in endometriosis patients. J Cell Physiol. 2018 Aug;233(8):5920-5925. doi: 10.1002/jcp.26401. Epub 2018 Feb 27. PMID: 29243819.

8. Khodaverdi S, Mohammadbeigi R, Khaledi M, Mesdaghinia L, Sharifzadeh F, Nasiripour S, Gorginzadeh M. Beneficial Effects of Oral Lactobacillus on Pain Severity in Women Suffering from Endometriosis: A Pilot Placebo-Controlled Randomized Clinical Trial. Int J Fertil Steril. 2019 Oct;13(3):178-183. doi:10.22074/ijfs.2019.5584.

Epub 2019 Jul 14. PMID: 31310070; PMCID: PMC6642422.

9. Schink M, Konturek PC, Herbert SL, Renner SP, Burghaus S, Blum S, Fasching PA, Neurath MF, Zopf Y. Different nutrient intake and prevalence of gastrointestinal comorbidities in women with endometriosis. J Physiol Pharmacol. 2019 Apr;70(2). doi: 10.26402/jpp.2019.2.09. Epub 2019 Aug 20. PMID: 31443088.

Manufactured by Amazon.ca
Bolton, ON